PECTUS EXCAVATUM SURGERY DIET

Nourishing Recovery And Empowering Your Health Journey To Promote Healing

DR LUCAS KAYCE

DISCLAIMER

This book about illness and nutrition is not meant to replace expert medical advice, diagnosis, or treatment; rather, it is meant purely for informational reasons. This book's content is founded on broad concepts and recommendations for managing diseases and nutrition.

Before adopting any major dietary or lifestyle changes, readers are recommended to speak with a qualified healthcare provider, such as a licensed physician or registered dietitian, especially if they have pre-existing medical concerns. Everybody has different health demands, so what works for one person might not work for another.

The use of the information provided in this book may have unfavorable repercussions or consequences, for which the author and publisher disclaim all liability. No disease is meant to be identified, treated, cured, or prevented by the information provided.

The book may include contain references to medical literature or research findings; however readers are urged to independently confirm this material and contact reliable sources.

It is important to remember that the fields of nutrition and medicine are always changing, and that new findings could have an impact on the advice offered in this book. As a result, readers are urged to keep up with the most recent advancements in healthcare and, when in doubt, seek professional counsel.

By reading this book, readers agree that they are in charge of their own health decisions and release the author and publisher from any liability arising from the use of the material in the book, whether direct or indirect.

TABLE OF CONTENTS

ABOUT THE BOOK

For those undergoing surgery for pectus excavatum, a disorder marked by a sunken chest, the book "Pectus Excavatum Surgery Diet" provides a thorough guide. The complexity of pectus excavatum, its etiology, and its effects on day-to-day living make this work extremely important. One of the main topics is how surgery is used to treat this illness and, most importantly, how important food is to the healing process.

The book explain what patients need to do in terms of preoperative care, covering not only the medical and psychological elements but also the critical significance that lifestyle modifications and the maintenance of a healthy diet play. It is essential to comprehend the surgical method, and the book provides a thorough examination of pectus excavatum surgery, covering a range of techniques, dangers, advantages, and expectations following the procedure.

The important post-surgery phase is the subject of the next chapters, which concentrate on nutrition in particular. The book carefully describes the post-operative diet to follow, the phased return to solid foods, and the necessary nutrients for the healing process. The creation of a healing meal plan is covered in detail, with special attention paid to the significance of protein consumption, vital nutrients, water, and foods to stay away from while recovering.

Acknowledging the readers' practical requirements, the book goes beyond theory by offering doable fixes. It provides a variety of recovery-focused dishes, such as nutritious smoothies, soothing soups, soft and simple-to-digest meals, and quick-energy snack options. The book also discusses difficulties that arise after surgery, including dietary limitations, stomach problems, taste changes, and swings in hunger, and it offers doable solutions for these problems.

Most importantly, the book offers long-term advice by examining how to gradually resume a regular diet, keep up a healthy lifestyle, keep an eye on nutritional requirements, and engage in physical exercise after surgery. This book is a priceless resource that offers a comprehensive approach to pectus excavatum surgery recovery, arming readers with the information and resources they require for fruitful and long-lasting recuperation.

RECOGNIZING THE PECTUS EXCAVATUM

The abnormal inward displacement of the sternum and ribs is a characteristic of Pectus Excavatum, a congenital abnormality of the chest wall. The appearance of a "sunken chest" or concave is produced by this indentation. Pectus Excavatum, often known as funnel chest, is commonly observed in childhood or adolescence as the chest wall development becomes more noticeable. Although the precise causation of this disorder is still unknown, it is generally acknowledged to have several origins that are influenced by both environmental and hereditary variables. While a genetic component has been found in certain cases, the exact genetic pathways causing Pectus Excavatum are currently being studied.

EFFECTS ON DAY-TO-DAY LIVING

Pectus excavatum has an effect on daily living that goes beyond its outward appearance. In addition to possible aesthetic issues, people with this illness may have cardiovascular and pulmonary consequences. Breathlessness, chest pain, and a decreased ability to tolerate physical exertion can result from the compression of essential organs including the heart and lungs. The visual abnormality may hurt one's body image and self-esteem, especially during adolescence, a crucial time for identity formation. This has important psychosocial ramifications as well.

SURGERY'S PLACE IN TREATMENT

When it comes to Pectus Excavatum treatment, surgery frequently has a big impact on both the functional and aesthetic aspects. The degree of the deformity, the patient's age, and the existence of concomitant symptoms all play a role in the decision to have surgery. The Nuss operation, which gradually reshapes the chest wall by placing a metal bar beneath the sternum, is the most common surgical intervention. This process has demonstrated efficacy in enhancing Pectus excavatum's physiological function as well as its outward appearance.

DIET IS IMPORTANT FOR RECOVERY AFTER PECTUS EXCAVATUM SURGERY

The need for postoperative care cannot be emphasized, even though surgery is an essential part of treatment. Following Pectus Excavatum surgery, recovery calls for a multifaceted strategy, with nutrition playing a critical part. To promote healing, tissue repair, and general recovery, proper nutrition is crucial. A balanced diet boosts the immune system, lowers the chance of problems, and speeds up the healing process. After Pectus Excavatum surgery, patients recover more quickly when they consume foods high in nutrients, stay hydrated, and follow any dietary advice given by medical professionals.

Comprehending Pectus Excavatum necessitates a multifaceted viewpoint that includes its definition, causes, effects on day-to-day functioning, the function of surgery in treatment, and the significance of nutrition in the recuperation process. Continued efforts to identify the many genetic and environmental factors that contribute to Pectus excavatum may lead to more tailored interventions and better outcomes for those who are afflicted with the disorder as medical science develops.

CHAPTER ONE

GETTING READY FOR SURGERY

MEDICAL ASSESSMENT AND ADVICE

A thorough medical evaluation and consultation are essential steps in the preparation process before surgery. To evaluate the patient's general health and make sure they are physically ready for the treatment, this stage is crucial for the medical staff as well as the patient. A detailed review of the patient's past medical history, current prescriptions, and any pre-existing medical issues is usually included in the evaluation. Finding possible dangers and complications that can occur before or after surgery is made easier with the use of this information.

Additionally, the consultation gives the patient a chance to speak candidly with their healthcare professional and ask any questions or voice any worries they may have regarding the upcoming medical procedure. By working together, medical practitioners can customize the surgical technique to the patient's unique demands and circumstances.

PSYCHOLOGICAL READINESS

Surgery can be a psychologically taxing procedure, thus psychological readiness is critical to a successful outcome. Before surgery, patients frequently experience emotional tension and worry, and it is critical to treat these issues for the patient's overall well-being. To assist patients in overcoming anxiety or nervousness, healthcare professionals may provide counseling or other forms of support. Psychological stress can be considerably reduced by having a clear understanding of the process, possible results, and expectations following surgery.

Furthermore, patients are urged to discuss any worries or problems they may be having honestly and openly with their medical staff. Psychological preparation includes building a transparent and supportive relationship between the patient and medical staff, which can enhance the surgery experience overall.

MODIFICATIONS IN LIFESTYLE BEFORE SURGERY

To improve their health and increase the likelihood of a successful outcome, people may be encouraged to adopt particular lifestyle adjustments in the weeks or months preceding surgery. A few examples of these adjustments are dietary adjustments, consistent exercise regimens, and giving up bad habits like smoking or binge drinking. Engaging in regular physical activity can lead to better recovery outcomes and cardiovascular health. It's imperative to give up smoking because it can hinder the body's healing process and raise the possibility of problems. Following these lifestyle changes creates the groundwork for long-term well-being as well as contributes to the effectiveness of the surgery.

THE VALUE OF A WELL-BALANCED DIET

A well-rounded and nourishing diet is essential for both facilitating the best possible recovery and getting the body ready for surgery.

Eating a range of nutrients, such as proteins, minerals, and vitamins, helps the body fight off infections and recover itself. Patients are frequently instructed to keep up a diet high in healthy grains, fruits, and vegetables as well as lean proteins. Sufficient fluid intake is equally important for several body processes and can help avoid issues like dehydration when recovering. In addition, maintaining a healthy diet before surgery strengthens the body's resistance, making it more capable of enduring the strain and requirements of the impending surgery. Healthcare professionals frequently offer dietary advice to tailor nutritional recommendations according to the specific needs of each patient and the type of surgery being performed.

CHAPTER TWO

THE PROCEDURE OF SURGERY

AN OVERVIEW OF SURGERY ON PECTUS EXCAVATUM

A congenital condition where the chest seems sunken or hollowed can be corrected with pectus excavatum surgery, sometimes referred to as chest wall reconstruction. This disorder, called pectus excavatum, can affect a person's respiratory, cardiac, and self-esteem in addition to causing them to feel physically and psychologically uncomfortable. Reshaping the chest wall to obtain a more symmetrical and natural appearance is part of the surgical procedure that will ultimately improve the patient's overall health.

SURGICAL PROCEDURE TYPES

Plectus excavatum is treated surgically using a variety of techniques, each according to the patient's unique requirements and the degree of the deformity. A popular surgery that uses a curved metal rod to elevate the sternum and remodel the chest is called the Nuss procedure. As an alternative, the Ravitch technique entails more involved surgery when the deformity is corrected by removing cartilage and ribs.

The severity of the pectus excavatum, the patient's age, and general health all have a role in the procedure that is chosen.

BENEFITS AND RISKS

Pectus excavatum surgery has inherent risks and potential advantages like any other surgical procedure. Adverse reactions to anesthesia, hemorrhage, or infection are examples of complications that highlight the significance of careful preoperative evaluations and aftercare. However, the operation frequently has major side effects as well, treating the psychological as well as the physical parts of the problem. Among the benefits that patients may encounter is better cardiac and respiratory health, improved physical appearance, and heightened self-esteem.

AFTER SURGERY ANTICIPATIONS

Expectations following surgery are essential to the procedure's overall success. The length of recovery varies based on the kind of surgery done and how well the patient responds to it. Following surgery, patients should generally anticipate some discomfort, edema, and bruising; however, these side effects usually go away with time.

It's imperative to schedule follow-up visits with medical specialists to track advancement and handle any issues that can surface throughout the recuperation phase. At first, physical activity could be limited, but as the patient recovers, a gradual return to regular daily activities and exercise is advised.

Pectus excavatum surgery is a difficult procedure meant to fix a congenital chest abnormality that might affect a person's physical and mental health. Patients contemplating or undergoing surgery must have a thorough understanding of the many surgical procedures available, as well as the related risks benefits, and expectations following the procedure. When combined with extensive pre-and postoperative care and advances in medical technology, pectus excavatum surgery can dramatically enhance the quality of life for those who suffer from this ailment.

CHAPTER THREE

AFTER SURGERY DIET

GUIDELINES FOR THE IMMEDIATE POST-OP DIET

Following surgery, following certain post-surgical dietary recommendations is an important part of the healing process. To promote the body's healing and reduce difficulties, careful consideration of food choices is necessary in the early postoperative time. Guidelines for the immediate post-operative diet usually call for a gradual return of food to allow the digestive tract to heal from the trauma of the procedure.

Patients are frequently instructed to begin with clear liquids in the early stages, such as broth, water, and clear juices. These liquids supply vital electrolytes and aid in preventing dehydration. The diet can be expanded to include full liquids such as yogurt, pudding, and pureed soups as soon as the patient can handle these.

The gastrointestinal tract can restore function and adjust to the return of various textures and consistencies thanks to this progressive approach.

PROGRESSIVE TRANSITION TO SOLID FOODS

It takes time and consideration for each person's tolerance levels to go from eating liquid to solid foods. Typically, the shift to more easily digested foods like mashed potatoes, soft vegetables, and lean proteins happens first. Initially, chewing can be difficult, so choosing softer textures facilitates simpler digestion. It's critical to keep an eye on how the body reacts to each diet phase and make adjustments based on tolerance and comfort level.

THE NEED FOR A PROPER DIET TO PROMOTE HEALING

The needs regarding nutrition are crucial to the healing process following surgery. Consuming enough protein is especially crucial since it promotes tissue healing and preserves muscle mass. Antioxidants, zinc, and vitamin

C are among the nutrients that boost the immune system and lower inflammation, which helps in the healing process. It is essential to keep up a diet that is well-balanced and rich in different vitamins and minerals to promote general healing and avoid nutritional deficiencies.

NUTRITIONAL GUIDELINES FOR THE MANAGEMENT OF PAIN

Another important component of post-surgery care is pain control, and diet can help with this. Due to their anti-inflammatory qualities, some foods can help with pain and swelling reduction. Flaxseeds and fatty fish, which are high in omega-3 fatty acids, are well known for their anti-inflammatory properties. Consuming foods high in antioxidants, such as fruits and vegetables, can also aid in the fight against oxidative stress, which is frequently increased throughout the healing process.

Staying hydrated is essential for recovering from surgery as well as continuing rehabilitation. A well-hydrated body facilitates detoxification and promotes general healing. People must consume enough fluids, taking into account things like the kind of surgery, their health, and any particular advice from medical professionals.

Nutrition following surgery is critical to the healing process. Ensuring a successful recovery requires adhering to immediate post-operative diet instructions, progressively transitioning to solid foods, and fulfilling nutritional needs for healing. Including food advice for pain management can also help promote a more comfortable and successful recovery. As always, personalized guidance from medical experts is essential to customizing the post-surgery dietary regimen to unique requirements and situations.

CHAPTER FOUR

CREATING A REMEDY DIET PLAN

THE SIGNIFICANCE OF CONSUMING PROTEIN

Consuming protein is essential for creating a healing diet plan because it is necessary for the body's tissues to mend and regenerate. The creation of hormones, enzymes, and other substances involved in the healing process depends on proteins. Consuming enough protein helps boost immune system function and repair damaged tissues, which makes it especially crucial during the healing phase following disease or injury. Incorporating lean protein sources like fish, chicken, beans, and tofu will help facilitate a quicker and more efficient recovery.

INCLUDING CRUCIAL NUTRIENTS

A complete healing diet plan must include critical nutrients in addition to protein. Antioxidants, vitamins, and minerals are examples of essential nutrients that are necessary for several physiological processes. For example, vitamins C and E support the body's defenses against inflammation and oxidative damage. Immune system performance and tissue repair are aided by minerals like magnesium and zinc. A well-rounded supply of vital nutrients is ensured by including a variety of fruits, vegetables, whole grains, and nuts in the diet, which supports the body's healing processes.

HYDRATION: AN ESSENTIAL PART OF HEALING

It is impossible to overestimate the importance of hydration as a component of any rehabilitation plan. Water is necessary for many biological processes, such as the transportation of nutrients, the regulation of body temperature, and the removal of waste.

Maintaining good blood circulation is essential for supplying nutrients and oxygen to cells involved in the healing process, and being appropriately hydrated helps achieve this. Dehydration can make recovery more difficult by interfering with these vital functions. To promote hydration throughout the healing phase, it is advised to drink lots of water, herbal teas, and electrolyte-rich liquids.

FOODS NOT TO EAT WHILE RECOVERING

Just as important as deciding what to include in a healing diet is thinking about what to avoid while recovering from an illness. Sugary snacks, highly processed foods, and excessive coffee or alcohol consumption can all hinder the healing process. These things could aggravate inflammation, weaken the immune system, and obstruct the body's ability to absorb nutrients.

Furthermore, some foods—like those heavy in refined carbohydrates or saturated fats—may make pre-existing medical issues worse. Reducing or avoiding certain foods can help to create a more healing and recuperative atmosphere.

Creating a healing diet plan entails considering the significance of protein consumption for tissue repair, including a range of vital nutrients for general health, realizing the importance of hydration for the healing process, and being aware of foods that could obstruct healing. A nutrient-rich, well-balanced diet is the best way for people to provide their bodies with the resources they need to heal quickly and return to optimal health.

CHAPTER FIVE

REMEDY RECIPES

SOFT AND EASY-TO-DIGEST FOODS

Including soft and easy-to-digest foods in your diet can be crucial for decreasing digestive stress and supporting healing during the recovery phase. Usually, the items in these meals are easy on the stomach and simple for the body to digest. Go for lean proteins like boiled chicken or tofu, steamed veggies, and well-cooked grains like rice and quinoa. Sweet potatoes or mashed potatoes make great alternatives as well. Steer clear of meals that are too seasoned, oily, or spicy to avoid causing your digestive tract extra discomfort. For additional nutritional value, think about adding fats that are simple to digest, such as olive oil.

SMOOTHIES AND SHAKES PACKED WITH NUTRIENTS

These nutrient-dense drinks are a flexible and easy method to provide your body with the vitamins and minerals it needs to heal. These drinks can be altered to meet dietary requirements and personal tastes. Add a range of fruits, including mangoes, bananas, and berries, as well as leafy greens like kale or spinach. Protein powder or Greek yogurt are two examples of sources of protein that can be used to improve nutritional value and facilitate muscle recovery.

For more hydration, think about adding beverages like coconut water or almond milk. Rich in nutrients, smoothies and shakes are not only good for your general health but also a convenient and reviving choice for people who aren't feeling very hungry.

REMEDY BROTHS & SOUPS

For many years, people have acknowledged the calming and nourishing qualities of healing soups and broths, which makes them the perfect option for those undergoing rehabilitation. Select nutritious broth-based soups that are high in minerals, vitamins, and other nutrients. Particularly chicken soup is a time-tested cure that is well-known for its ability to lessen cold and flu symptoms. Vegetable broth or miso soup are good vegetarian substitutes that can be just as healthy. To improve the nutritional profile, add whole grains, lean meats, and a range of veggies.

In addition to being soothing, the soup's warmth promotes hydration and facilitates easier digestion. Healing soup consumption can be a reassuring custom that enhances general well-being while in recovery.

SNACK IDEAS TO GET YOU STARTED FAST

Snacks are essential for sustaining energy levels during the healing process. Snacking on foods high in nutrients can give the body a rapid and effective source of energy. For a well-balanced energy boost, think about snacking on protein, healthy fats, and carbohydrates.

Some great ideas are a handful of nuts and dried fruits, Greek yogurt with honey and berries, or nut butter on wholegrain crackers. Energy bars with a combination of nuts, seeds, and dried fruits can also be easy to carry with you as a quick snack.

Drinking water or herbal teas with food can improve general well-being because both are crucial for hydration. Not only are these easy, high-energy snacks tasty, but they also help promote a gradual, pain-free recuperation.

CHAPTER SIX

OVERCOMING OBSTACLES

HANDLING NUTRITIONAL LIMITATIONS

Managing dietary restrictions can be very difficult, requiring people to choose their food intake carefully and intelligently. Dietary limits necessitate a greater understanding of nutritional requirements, regardless of whether they are imposed by medical issues, allergies, or personal preferences.

This frequently entails reading labels carefully, closely examining ingredients, and organizing meals creatively. Overcoming dietary restrictions can be a life-changing experience that helps people develop a more sophisticated awareness of their nutritional needs and a flexible and varied palate.

People can use dietary restrictions as a springboard for creative cooking and better health by experimenting with substitute ingredients and learning new recipes.

HANDLING DIGESTIVE PROBLEMS

Digestive problems can be extremely difficult for a person's general health, affecting both their physical and mental well-being. Taking charge of your digestive health requires you to make several dietary and lifestyle changes in addition to getting the right medical advice. People who are aware of the patterns and triggers of digestive distress can make more informed decisions by including meals high in fiber, drinking enough water, and engaging in mindful eating. In certain instances, seeking advice from medical experts could be required to identify and treat underlying digestive issues, resulting in customized treatment regimens and improved quality of life.

HANDLING MODIFICATIONS IN FLAVOR AND HUNGER

Modifications in flavor and hunger can be unsettling, impacting meal satisfaction and overall enjoyment. Taste perceptions might change due to several reasons, such as age, medicine, or medical treatments. Adapting to such changes calls for a more sophisticated strategy than just changing recipes. Trying new flavors, textures, and cooking methods might encourage people to rediscover the pleasure of eating. Regaining an appreciation for food may also be facilitated by learning new cuisines and practicing mindfulness while eating. A well-balanced and fulfilling diet can be ensured by seeking assistance from nutritionists or dietitians, who can offer tailored techniques to address changes in appetite and taste.

SEEKING ASSISTANCE FROM MEDICAL EXPERTS

Getting help from medical experts becomes essential while dealing with health issues to overcome hurdles. People can get individualized advice and treatment strategies by keeping lines of communication open with physicians, dietitians, and other experts. Healthcare providers can offer important advice on how to handle dietary limits, take care of digestive problems, and adjust to changes in appetite and taste. Frequent tests, consultations, and check-ups aid in tracking development and enabling the required modifications to guarantee the best possible health results. Working together with medical experts creates a feeling of collaboration in overcoming obstacles, enhancing general well-being, and enabling people to actively participate in their health.

CHAPTER SEVEN

RETURNING GRADUALLY TO A REGULAR DIET

A gradual transition back to a regular diet following surgery or an extended time of food restrictions is frequently an important part of long-term dietary considerations. To ensure that the digestive system can adjust to a wider variety of foods without experiencing any discomfort or issues, this transition should be handled carefully.

Reintroducing familiar foods gradually enables the body to adjust and aids in the identification of any triggers or intolerances that may have emerged during the healing process.

By giving people's eating habits a sense of normalcy again, this gradual restoration promotes psychological health in addition to helping with physical healing.

SUSTAINING A BALANCED AND HEALTHFUL LIFESTYLE

A balanced and healthful lifestyle is essential for long-term well-being. Beyond the initial post-operative period, people ought to make an effort to include a range of nutrient-dense foods in their regular meals. A variety of fruits, vegetables, whole grains, lean meats, and healthy fats are included in this. To minimize overconsumption and promote weight management, it is imperative to emphasize portion control and mindful eating. Maintaining a balanced diet consistently gives the body the nutrition it needs to support general health, bolster the immune system, and help avert further health problems.

KEEPING AN EYE ON NUTRITIONAL REQUIREMENTS

It takes constant attention to food preferences, lifestyle modifications, and individual health situations to monitor nutritional demands. Dietary programs can be customized to match individual needs with the support of healthcare specialists like nutritionists or dietitians who provide routine consultations. This customized strategy takes into account variables such as age, gender, degree of activity, and any current health issues. Regular evaluations of dietary consumption guarantee that people get enough vitamins, minerals, and other vital nutrients, reducing the possibility of deficiencies that could affect general health. Maintaining a healthy lifestyle largely involves modifying the diet in response to evolving nutritional needs.

INCLUDING EXERCISE FOLLOWING SURGERY

One of the most important things for long-term recovery and overall well-being after surgery is to include physical activity in the routine. Exercise improves cardiovascular health, builds muscle, and increases mobility in addition to helping one maintain a healthy weight. Starting with low-impact workouts and working your way up to more intense ones is crucial. Don't forget to consider the patient's physical condition and any limitations after the surgery.

Combining aerobic, strength, and flexibility training builds physical resilience and aids in the body's entire healing process. It is a component of a holistic approach to health.

Long-term dietary considerations cover a wide range of strategies for regaining and sustaining health following surgery. The progressive reintroduction of a regular diet, the focus on maintaining a healthy and balanced lifestyle, the continuous assessment of nutritional requirements, and the integration of appropriate physical activities all enhance the general welfare of persons during their recovery process.

www.ingramcontent.com/pod-product-compliance
Lightning Source LLC
Chambersburg PA
CBHW060820260726
48660CB00003B/1012